Reiki Third Degree

Master Manual

The Didactic Dimension Of The Universal Life Force

ANDREA SCARSI

DEDICATED

To The Reiki And Us Loving It

TABLE OF CONTENTS

NOTE OF THE AUTHOR

The Author strived to be as accurate and complete as possible in the creation of this book. Nevertheless, he affirms that the contents expressed in it are solely the result of his knowledge, experience, and personal understanding of the considered discipline. He does not guarantee and declare at any time that these are absolute and unequivocal.

While he made all attempts to verify the information provided in this publication, he assumes no responsibility for errors, omissions, interpretations, or experimentations of the subject matter herein.

Any perceived slights of specific persons, peoples, companies, or organizations are unintentional.

In self-help books and manuals, there are no guarantees of performed results or income made, as one expects—the Author caution the Readers to rely on their judgment about any circumstance and act accordingly.

This book does not pretend, in any way, to stand as an official professional source of any kind, be it medical, dietetic, psychological, religious, legal, commercial, accounting, or financial. The Readers are advised to seek the services of competent professionals in the abovementioned fields.

www.andreascarsi.com/english.htm.

ANDREA SCARSI

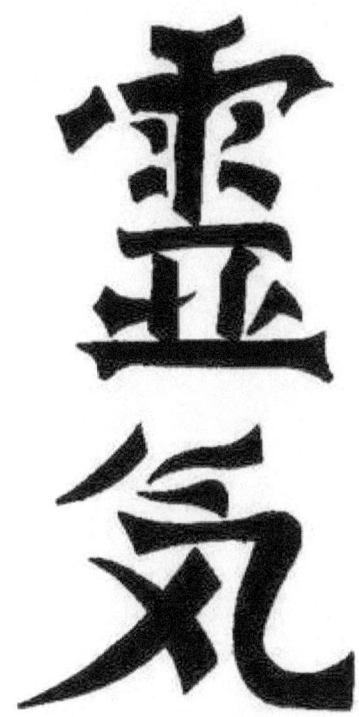

I thank the Reiki Master *Ma Advaita Krisana* for the drawing above.

INTRODUCTION

Welcome to the didactic dimension of Reiki, the Third and Master Degree Level. In this seminar, the fourth and final symbol of Reiki is transmitted and revealed to you, the Master Symbol, which allows you to open the Reiki channel and generate new lines of Reiki Operators.

You'll learn how to use it to activate all the Reiki levels, to give individual o group sessions as a Reiki Master, to propagate the technique, activate planetary places, and integrate the three levels of Reiki.

You are now a Reiki Master, and your responsibility is to keep yourself that.

Given the difficulty of language, as regards the masculine and feminine, since your Reiki students are going to be both male and female, I have adopted a language strategy to explain the initiating procedure as if you were alternatively activating, and attuning one and the other.

This is the manual that I give to my Reiki students upon completing the Third Level Master Seminar.

That's universal teaching.

Let's start.

ANDREA SCARSI

DAI KHOMYO

The Great Enlightenment

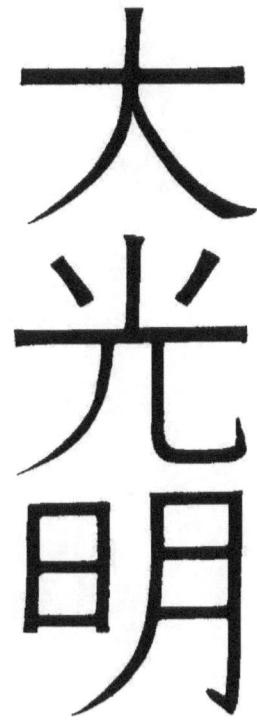

Dai Khòmyo opens the Reiki channel.

You draw it large with the palm of your hand, pronouncing it three times,

Dai Khòmyo,
Dai Khòmyo,
Dai Khòmyo,

Dai and Khòmyo are two Japanese words meaning, the first one, Great, and the second one, Enlightenment. (Khòmyo, meaning enlightenment, is composed of Kho, which means light, and Myo, which means wisdom, directly deriving from Sanskrit, when Buddhism reached Japan. It's however, just one word.)

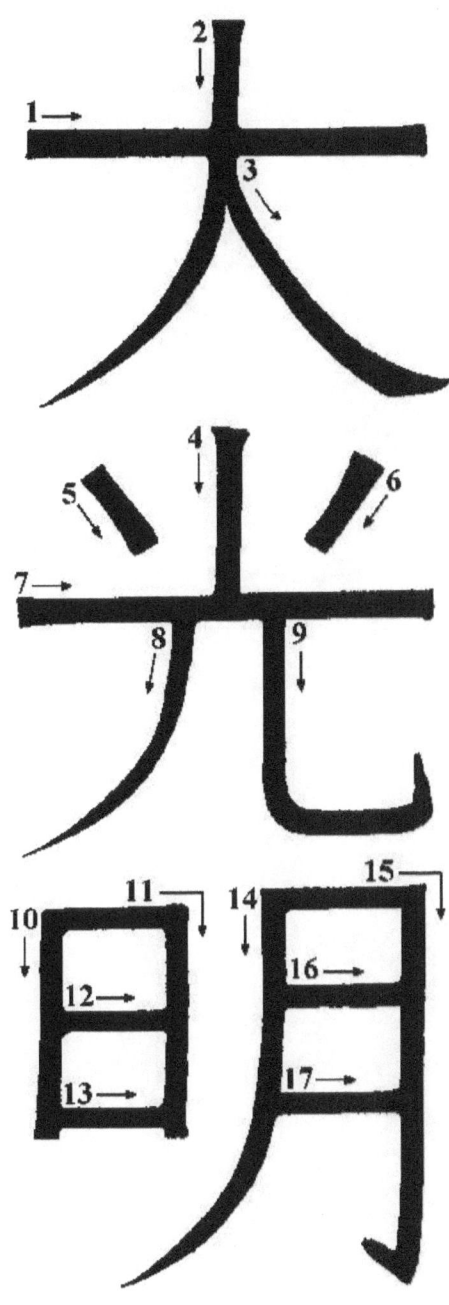

FIRST LEVEL INITIATION AND ATTUNEMENT PROCEDURE

FOUR ACTIVATIONS

Make conscious contact with your Reiki channel and open it. Activate your maximum flow of Reiki energy and start the activation for yourself and the place where you are performing the seminar. Silently call all four symbols in succession, drawing them large with your dominant hand, starting with DKM, then CKR, SHK, HSTSN.

You and the place get filled with Reiki.

Approach your student and stand behind him, making him partaker of your Reiki channel.

Let him enter your channel, your Reiki field of Universal Life Force, and energetically wrap him up, boost, accompany, and protect him.

Silently call the DKM on the top of his head, drawing it large on the aura, then transmit it in by placing your hand on his scalp.

Feel it creeping gently in, and opening the channel; feel it making its way and penetrate deeper and deeper, radiating, cleaning, and stimulating; more and more down to the Anahata and Muladhara.

Continue transmitting.

It'll progressively penetrate with each subsequent activation.

Then, one at a time, starting with the CKR, call the other three symbols on the top of his head, on the aura, and transmit them in, one by one, resting your hand on his scalp.

Perceive them gently creep along the channel; feel them making their way and deeply penetrate, transferring their specific energy and dimension, deeper and deeper until reaching the Anahata and Muladhara.

Continue transmitting.

They'll progressively penetrate with each subsequent activation.

Take, then, position in front of your student and activate his hands' chakras, at the center of his palms, one hand at a time, with a circular touch on the palm to bring there his attention.

Then, silently call all the symbols, one hand at a time, in his palm's aura and transmit them in, by placing your hand on his, and feel and visualize them flowing up to the Anahata and Sahasrara, and down to the Muladhara and legs.

Feel and observe, by your third eye, your and your student's Reiki channel merging and joining.

Then blow on his palms to push them further inside.

Activate the remaining six chakras, from sixth to first, blowing on them, to the front first, then behind.

Invite your student to lie down and activate, the same way, his feet's chakras, one foot at a time, with a circular touch on the sole.

Silently call all the symbols, one foot at a time, in his sole's aura and transmit them in, placing your hand on his foot sole, feeling and visualizing them slide along his legs up to the Muladhara, Anahata, and Sahasrara.

Feel and observe, by your third eye, how both your Reiki channels are merging and joining.

Then blow on his sole to push them further inside.

Move to your next student.

The work is complete.

Now close the activation for yourself, for the place, and for the work you've done, by drawing all symbols in reverse order with DKM last.

Clap your hands, move away, and let go.

ANDREA SCARSI

SECOND LEVEL INITIATION AND ATTUNEMENT PROCEDURE

FOUR ACTIVATIONS
ONE FOR EACH SYMBOL PLUS A COMPLETE ONE

Make conscious contact with your Reiki channel and open it. Activate your maximum flow of Reiki energy and start the activation for yourself and the place where you are performing the seminar. Silently call all four symbols in succession, drawing them large with your dominant hand, starting with DKM, then CKR, SHK, HSTSN.

You and the place get filled with Reiki.

Approach your student and stand behind her, making her partaker of your Reiki channel.

Let her enter your channel, your Reiki field of Universal Life Force, and energetically wrap her up, boost, accompany, and protect her.

Silently call the DKM on the top of her head, drawing it large on the aura, and then transmit it in by placing your hand on her scalp.

Feel it creeping gently in, and opening the channel; feel it making its way and penetrate deeper and deeper, radiating, cleaning, and stimulating; more and more down to the Anahata and Muladhara.

Continue transmitting.

It'll progressively penetrate with each subsequent activation.

Then, one at a time, starting with the CKR, silently call the other symbols, naming only the one you're teaching, on the top of her head, on the aura, and transmit them in, one by one, resting your hand on her scalp.

Perceive them gently creep along the channel; feel them making their way and deeply penetrate, transferring their specific energy and dimension, deeper and deeper until reaching the Anahata and Muladhara.

Continue transmitting.

They'll progressively penetrate with each subsequent activation.

Take, then, position in front of your student to activate her hands' chakras, at the center of her palms, one hand at a time.

Silently call all the symbols in the aura, one hand at a time, starting with DKM; name and draw on her palm, with one finger, only the symbol that you are teaching, to activate it to her consciousness, and then transmit them all inside placing your hand on hers.

Transmit. Feel and visualize them flowing up to the Anahata and Sahasrara, and down to the Muladhara and legs.

Feel and observe, by your third eye, your and your student's Reiki channel merging and joining.

Then blow on her palms to push them further inside.

Activate the remaining six chakras, silently calling and drawing in the Aura of each chakra the symbol that you are teaching. Pitch it and blow it in, to the front first, and then behind.

Invite your student to lie down and activate, the same way, his feet's chakras, one foot at a time.

Silently call all the symbols in the aura, one foot at a time, starting with DKM; name and draw on the center of her foot sole, with one finger, only the symbol that you are teaching, to activate it to her consciousness, and then transmit them all in placing your hand on her sole.

Transmit. Feel and visualize them flowing up her legs to the Muladhara and Anahata, along her arms and hands, and up to the Sahasrara.

Feel and observe, by your third eye, how both your Reiki channels are merging and joining.

Then blow on her sole to push them further inside.

Move to your next student.

The work is complete.

Now close the activation for yourself, for the place, and for the work you've done, by drawing all symbols in reverse order with DKM last.

Clap your hands, move away, and let go.

Now The Fourth Activation
Follow the procedure above but drawing and naming all the three symbols.

ANDREA SCARSI

THIRD LEVEL MASTER INITIATION AND ACTIVATION PROCEDURE

ONE ACTIVATION

Make conscious contact with your Reiki channel and open it. Activate your maximum flow of Reiki energy and start the activation for yourself and the place where you are performing the seminar. Silently call all four symbols in succession, drawing them large with your dominant hand, starting with DKM, then CKR, SHK, HSTSN.

You and the place get filled with Reiki.

Approach your student and stand behind him, making him partaker of your Reiki channel.

Let him enter your channel, your Reiki field of Universal Life Force, and energetically wrap him up, boost, accompany, and protect him.

Call and name the DKM on the top of his head, drawing it large on the aura, then transmit it in by placing your hand on his scalp.

Feel it creeping gently in, and opening the channel; feel it making its way and penetrate deeper and deeper, radiating, cleaning, and stimulating; more and more down to the Anahata and Muladhara.

Continue transmitting.

Then, one at a time, starting with the CKR, call and name the other three symbols on the top of her head, on the aura, and transmit them in, one by one, resting your hand on her scalp.

Perceive them gently creep along the channel; feel them making their way and deeply penetrate, transferring their specific energy and dimension, deeper and deeper until reaching the Anahata and Muladhara.

Continue transmitting.

Position yourself in front of the student and activate his hand's chakras, one at a time.

Draw the DKM with a finger on his palms, one at the time, and transmit it in, placing your hand on his hand.

Transmit and push it in; watch it and feel it flow along the meridians of his arms up to the heart and the Sahasrara, and down to the Muladhara, along the meridians of his legs, to his feet.

Feel and see how your channel and the student's one and the Reiki melt and unite you both.

Blow it further inside.

Draw and name then with your finger, one by one, the three sacred symbols on the palm of his hand starting with CKR and transmit them in. Feel and visualize them penetrate and run up along the meridians of his arms and reach the Anahata and Sahasrara, and down to the Muladhara, and the meridians of his legs to his feet.

Feel and see how your channel and the student one and the Reiki melt and unite you both.

Blow them further inside.

Activate the DKM in the remaining six chakras.

Call and name it in the Aura of each chakra and throw and blow it in, front and back.

Invite the student to lie down and activate the chakra of the feet, one at a time.

Draw and name the DKM on his plant with a finger and transmit it in. Visualize it flowing along the meridians of the legs up to the Muladhara, Anahata and Sahasrara and arms and hands.

Blow it further inside.

Draw and name then, one by one, the three symbols on the sole beginning with CKR and transmit them in; visualize them scroll to the Muladhara, Anahata, and Sahasrara and along the meridians of his legs, arms, and hands.

Feel and see how your channel, the student's, and the Reiki merge and unite you both.

The work is complete.

Now close the activation for you, the place and the work you have done by redesigning the symbols in reverse order, with DKM last.

Clap your hands and log off.

ANDREA SCARSI

TEACHING THE REIKI FIRST DEGREE

It requires four sessions, each including one attunement.

Explain the Reiki, practice the standard self-treatment, and perform the initial activation.

Explain the Chakras, practice the self-treatment, and treatment and run the second activation.

Explain the Standard Session and do practice the full treatment.

Explain the other types of session and do get the full treatment.

The training can take place on the weekend, in two separate days or four evenings.

There are no prerequisites.

TEACHING THE REIKI SECOND DEGREE

It requires four sessions, each comprehensive of one attunement.

Explain and practice the First Symbol and perform its first activation.

Explain and practice the Second Symbol and perform its second activation.

Explain and practice the Third Symbol and perform its third Activation.

Review the Symbols and integrate the First and Second Level in the Standard Session.

The training can take place on the weekend, in two separate days or four evenings.

Prerequisites: Reiki First Degree and ten sessions of practice.

ANDREA SCARSI

TEACHING THE REIKI THIRD MASTER DEGREE

It requires four separate sessions and one attunement.

Review the First Level.

Review the Second Level.

Explain the MASTER symbol, and when you feel, run the activation.

Explain the procedures of teaching.

Make a practice of the Master Symbol.

Make a practice of the activation of the three levels.

Integrate the First, Second, and Master levels in Standard Session.

The training can take place on the weekend, in two separate days or four evenings.

Prerequisites: Reiki Second Degree and ten sessions of practice.

ANDREA SCARSI

INTEGRATING THE THREE REIKI DEGREES

Integrate the Master Level with the First and Second levels and add the DKM symbol in your regular session.

DKM opens the channel Reiki.

You can use it in any position and at any time during your session work because it works well for specific situations and the local Reiki flow of organs and meridians.

When you feel that the flow is not activated or flows very slowly, call CKR or DKM.

Before each treatment and self-treatment, start the procedure of activation, begin channeling, center in our heart, and place your hands.

Call DKM on each position, along with CKR, SHK, and HSZSN, when you feel that is conducive to the maximum energy thrust.

Call it on the palm of your hands, along with CKR, SHK, and HSZSN, before starting your treatments, to activate your maximum Reiki flow.

On the crown position, during your treatments or self-treatment, call the DKM before or after SHK. It renews or prepares the activation.

At the end of each session, as the last act, call all the Symbols on the Aura and transmit them gently with a couple of passes, to complement, seal, and protect your work, in space and time.

Clap your hands and log off.

This Session has the value that you give it. Reiki is free; people contribute to the commitment, effort, resources, and time that you spent to learn and master the technique, to close the Reiki deal and be free to come again when they want.

CONCLUSIONS

You are now able to generate new channels Reiki.

Realize that your learning as a Reiki Master is complete when you have experienced the attunement of each of the three Reiki levels: First, Second, and Master.

No matter the sequence.

My suggestion is to talk about your mastery to friends and acquaintances; to let people know that you are a Reiki Master and share with them your experience and what can be shared.

Reiki takes its course and students will come to you when you go to them.

To further expand your practice - in addition to word of mouth - a great way to make yourself known is the use of leaflets, lectures, articles, and speeches on radio, television, and social networks you attend.

Also, whenever the situation comes, such as for parties and meetings, you can provide a short Reiki demonstration and distribute your business cards.

When people tell you they have trouble, introduce yourself, give a short treatment on the spot, five to ten minutes, and explains what Reiki is and does. It's always good publicity, and you can distribute your business cards.

Welcoming students who have received an attunement from other Reiki Masters, the best approach is quick quality control and asking to see their diplomas. It indicates seriousness and professionalism on your part.

Plus give them your corresponding manuals.

In case anyone wishes to repeat a level with you, which he attended with another Reiki Master, you can ask half the cost, and they now go under your responsibility and protection.

When your students want to repeat a level with you, they can freely participate or contribute with an offer, and assist you.

If you do your job well, they ask you to repeat because of affection towards you.

As a Reiki Master, you are responsible for your students.

That means keeping yourself evolving, being centered, and available in your role.

It also means you help them stay on track, encouraging them to continue to practice.

When organizing Reiki exchanges or group sessions, always open the event with a general activation of participants and location.

I transmitted the Reiki from the line I descend, which teaches it as a spiritual practice and meditation, where the healing comes as a result of the harmony of the soul.

The ultimate healing is the freedom from all identifications, attachments, and limitations of the ego, thereby achieving enlightenment.

Reiki has no limits and travels on that dimension.

You can find differences with other Reiki Masters who teach it only as a technique for physical healing. That depends on their level of development.

We all do our best and travel at the speed that we are capable of.

Reiki is universal.

The best teaching strategy is one where you share your experience.

If you transmit information that you have not yet checked, just let it be known to our students and verify them soon.

It is good practice to keep a chronology of your activations, to remember at what level your students are and also to send then, now and then, a Reiki hug.

Lastly, do remember that the DKM is assimilated and integrated fully into your system over the next 21 days.

I invite you to practice daily for this period, whenever you remember, to become one with it.

Good job and have fun.

Andrea Scarsi

ANDREA SCARSI

ACTIVATING PLANETARY PLACES

When you open a Reiki attunement initiation, you're also activating the place where this takes place. You do it mainly to prepare for the subsequent activation of a student, yet you are activating the site.

That's why you can practice the activation procedure to activate a specific location and open a channel on the planet. When you feel it's required, or you have to do it or love to do it, or you want to donate Reiki, or seal an important event in our life, do it.

Remember the sites you're activating, always keep them present to your consciousness, and as a result, you can connect with them, wherever you are, via the third symbol and share your Reiki, joy, and gratitude.

MY MASTER GENEALOGY

Andrea Scarsi
Anand Mandira
Prem Aurelio
Deva Piaso
Nancy Morgan
Barbara Weber Ray
Hawayo Takata
Chujiro Hayashi
Mikao Usui

BIBLIOGRAPHY

Scarsi, Andrea 2012: The Secret Of Metaphysical Science
Scarsi, Andrea 2012: The Secret Of Meditation
Scarsi, Andrea 2013: Seeds Of Enlightenment
Scarsi, Andrea 2014: Reiki First Degree Manual
Scarsi, Andrea 2014: Reiki Second Degree Manual
Scarsi, Andrea 2014: Pearls of Wisdom

ABOUT THE AUTHOR

Dr. Andrea Scarsi, also known as Sandesh, is a master of silence and chaos. He defines himself as a mystic, metaphysician, author, musician, and wellness coach when he uses his works to share a dimension of being, lifestyle, and knowledge, founded on meditation and communion with the absolute.

The rest of the time, he lets himself go into life and enjoys what happens in the unified field of Awareness.

In the Osho Commune, he received his first Reiki session in 1988 in Poona, India. In the following years, he continued the practice and completed the learning of all three levels.

He became a Master Reiki on February 19, 1997, in Mahabaleshwar, Maharashtra, India, at 6.00 am, and is the ninth on Usui's genealogy line. At the moment, he activated 25 Reiki Masters.

Born in Venice, Italy, in 1955, he began practicing yoga and spiritism and experimenting with telepathy at fifteen. At eighteen, following a near-death experience, he contacts alien and transdimensional entities. At twenty-four, on his first trip to India, he finds himself a vegetarian and in the world of meditation led by India and the Spiritual Master Osho, receiving Sandesh as a new name, which he wears in specific environments.

He's often traveled, especially to India, residing for long periods also in Nepal, the Philippines, and Buddhist Southeast Asia: Japan, Thailand, Sri Lanka, Hong Kong, Laos, China, and Tibet, exploring out of curiosity and personal research, local places, and cultures, meeting people and participating in ritual and religious practices.

Over time, he deepens various meditative techniques for awakening consciousness, energy rebalancing, and personal evolution, which he practices and teaches by conducting groups, sessions, conferences, and songs.

He studied philosophy, earned a Ph.D. in Metaphysical Science, and various diplomas such as Holistic Life Coach, Reiki Grand Master, Master of Crystals, Shamanism, Meditation and Massage, and Wellness.

In 1991 he married Krisana and lives in Venice.

He's reachable at www.andreascarsi.com/english.htm.

BOOKS BY ANDREA SCARSI

Answers For The Soul: Fragments of Eternal Wisdom
Blessings! Dedicated to Osho
Extraterrestrial Channeling: Alien Abduction Syndrome
Happy To Be Happy: The Grand Manual Of Happiness
Home Sweet Home Staging: Easy Is Right
How To Ask A Woman Out: Gentlemen Only
Indigo Crystal Rainbow and Diamond: Tell Themselves
Journey To The Underworld: First Level Shamanic Procedures Manual
Make Your Own Vineyard: Ex Vite Vita
O Iguana! My Iguana! Herbivore is Beautiful
Pearls of Wisdom: Tales of Ordinary Metaphysics
Reiki First Degree Manual
Reiki Second Degree Manual
Reiki Third Degree Manual
Seeds Of Enlightenment: The Buddha Within
Tarot Reading Essentials: The New Basic Meaning Manual
The Art of Persuasion: How to Achieve Your Goals Ethically
The Art of Worrying: How to Enter and Exit it at Will
The Master And The Assassin: An Ordinary Zen Story
The Secret Of Meditation: The Inner Dimension
The Secret Of Metaphysical Science: Our Eternal Journey Through Infinite
Vegetarian Cuisine: Reasons Objections Recipes
Walking The Dogs: A Dialogue A Manual
Zen The Sense Of Nonsense: Anecdotes For Synaptic Deprogramming

MANTRAS BY ANDREA SCARSI (SANDESH)

Mantras Mahamantras
The Mantra Experiment
The Mantra Way
Om Namo Supernova
Amavasya

A mantra is a Verbal Being acting as a bridge between the human and the divine. It carries our prayer, thankfulness, and gratitude and is an entity in its own right. When we recite or sing it to communicate with the superior dimension, in addition to words and sound, we also employ intention, energy, devotion, and focus. All this raises us immediately. It increases our emotional state and makes us touch God.

A mantra is an introspective event turning to the multiple aspects of the One by evoking its symbolic names: Shiva, Brahma, Vishnu, Ganesha, Laxmi, Saraswati, Gurudev, and Shanti; names representing the infinite manifestation of the cosmic cycle. They are magic formulas for amending the universal present, resolving the apparent fragmentation, and recreating the union of consciousness with what is.

A mantra is to be recited and sung without interruption to convey the intact message, and breathing comes between recitations. Let's get lost in the mantra, and let the vehicle, the human, and the divine become one. That's the power of the mantra. We recite it and go deeper until melting what we were before, our intention, recitation, sound, and collective energy, and manifesting unity once again, the yoga of consciousness, the absolute presence, whose supreme name is Om.

BOOKS BY ANDREA SCARSI IN ITALIAN

21 Giorni: Diario di un Ritiro Spirituale

A Proposito di Osho: Conferenze di Un Suo Discepolo

Benedizioni!: Dedicato a Osho

Benvenuti ad Atlantide: Cristalli e Chakra Riequilibrio di Primo Livello

Breve Storia Dei Sogni: Nella Visione Occidentale

Canalizzazioni Extraterrestri: Sindrome da Rapimento Alieno

Casa Dolce Casa Vendesi: Home Staging Facile

Dhyana Yoga: Unione Con L'Essenza

Dispense Reiki Primo Livello

Dispense Reiki Secondo Livello

Dispense Reiki Terzo Livello Master

Felici Di Essere Felici: Il Grande Manuale Della Felicità

Guarire Il Sé Ombra: Aneddoti Di Alleggerimento Di Carico

Il Lato Positronico: Ridondanze Di Un Androide

Il Maestro e l'Assassino: Una Consueta Storia Zen

Il Segreto della Meditazione: La Dimensione Interiore

Il Segreto della Scienza Metafisica: Il Nostro Eterno Viaggio nell'Infinito

Il Silenzio dell'Assoluto: Satsang con Sandesh

Immagina: E Accelera la Tua Crescita Personale

Indaco Cristallo Arcobaleno e Diamante: Si Raccontano

La Cucina Vegetariana: Motivazioni Obiezioni Ricette

L'Arte della Persuasione: Come Raggiungere Eticamente i Propri Obiettivi

L'Arte della Preoccupazione: Come Entrarci e Uscirne a Piacere

L'Arte di Cambiare: Modella la Tua Vita

L'Arte di Invitare una Donna: Solo per Gentiluomini

Le Compatibilità Zodiacali: Trova l'Anima Gemella con l'Astrologia

Lettura dei Tarocchi: Manuale dei Significati di Base

Massaggio Olistico: Manuale delle Procedure di Base

Menando Il Can Per L'Aia: Un Dialogo Un Manuale
Notiziario Reiki: Delle Attività Mensili Svolte
Perle di Saggezza: Racconti di Ordinaria Metafisica
Risposte per l'Anima: Frammenti di Eterna Saggezza
Semi di Illuminazione: Il Buddha Interiore
Transizione Vegetariana: Pe La Pecora Che Si Crede Leone
Viaggio nel Mondo di Sotto: Manuale di Procedura Sciamanica di Primo Livello
Zen Il Senso del Non Senso: Aneddoti di Deprogrammazione Sinaptica

You've reached the end of
Reiki Master Third Degree Manual

Thank You For Reading
Andrea Scarsi

This is the handbook that I give to my Reiki students after
their Third Degree Master Seminar, which lasts sixteen hours
(4x4) and is inclusive of one activation.

www.ingramcontent.com/pod-product-compliance
Lightning Source LLC
Chambersburg PA
CBHW051404280526
45784CB00007B/3085